The Integrative Relaxation Technique In Relaxation Therapy

By
Dr C.B.Ramachander
BABCP accredited Integrative Clinical Psychotherapist

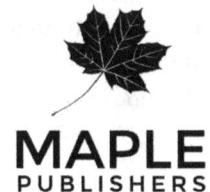

MAPLE
PUBLISHERS

The Integrative Relaxation Technique In Relaxation Therapy

Author: Dr C.B.Ramachander

Copyright © 2026 Dr C.B.Ramachander

The right of Dr C.B.Ramachander to be identified as author of this work has been asserted by the author in accordance with section 77 and 78 of the Copyright, Designs and Patents Act 1988.

First Published in 2026

ISBN 978-1-83538-785-6 (Paperback)
     978-1-83538-786-3 (E-Book)

Book Cover and Layout by:
    Maple Publishers

Published by:
    Maple Publishers
    Fairbourne Drive, Atterbury,
    Milton Keynes,
    MK10 9RG, UK
    www.maplepublishers.com

The views expressed in this work are solely those of the author and do not reflect the opinions of Publishers, and the Publisher hereby disclaims any responsibility for them. This book should not be used as a substitute for the advice of a competent authority, admitted or authorized to advise on the subjects covered.

A CIP catalogue record for this title is available from the British Library.

Dr. C.B. Ramachander

MBBS MSC (MHS) FRSPH BABCP
Accredited Cognitive Behavioural Psychotherapist

Postgraduate Diploma in clinical Psychotherapy

Diploma in Eating Disorders Practitioner skills (NCFED)

Diploma in Psychoanalysis

Diploma in EMDR Therapy

CONTENTS

Acknowledgment 5

Introduction 7

1. Relaxation – Definition Simplified 14
2. Integration – Leading to Innovation 15
3. Integrative Relaxation Technique 16
4. The Autonomic Nervous System and Psychophysiology of SDB 17
5. The Integrative Technique in Relaxation Therapy . 22
6. Positive Self Affirmations Statement 25
7. Conclusion 27

Acknowledgements

Although I have long continued to have an interest in writing on chosen topics, in my medical speciality of psychiatry and psychotherapy, due to work pressures and other excuses, I was unable to find the drive needed to write. It was my late wife, who passed away quite recently, who was my initial source of encouragement, always suggesting that I should put pen to paper she was always there to support me, in life she was "my rock."

Inspired, I recently decided to start writing, encouraged and persuaded by my son and his wife who have always been a great support and comfort to me.

Encouragement has come from many quarters, and from One and all (including my friends and work Colleagues) who I have always considered as friends.

And so, in my activities contributing to good standing, I decided to devote more time to book writing, under the heading of professional activities. Now finished, it is my hope that these books will become useful to a wide audience.

Special thanks go to Dr Mutiboko, Consultant Psychiatrist, who is my referee and is a person who has always encouraged me. Thanks also to Mr Tarn Maley, my close friend and author who gave me that extra push to start writing.

My heartfelt thanks to one and all, without whom this book may never have been written.

Introduction

I am a medical graduate. Initially, for a few years, I worked in India as a tutor in Pathology. Whilst there, I then became a chest physician, and Tuberculosis Medical officer.

Later, in 1974, I decided to come to England where I trained as a psychiatrist. With devoted interest, I advanced at different levels within this field and worked as a consultant psychiatrist for a number of years.

After my retirement from the NHS in 2008, I worked as a locum consultant psychiatrist and have a great interest in psychotherapy. I have developed this interest and have become well qualified in this field.

From 29.07.2025, I have decided to develop and establish more interest and further developments in the field of psychotherapy. I have also established my own website in psychotherapy services for the public (https://www.dr-ramachanders-psychotherapy-service.com). I will be concentrating on relapse prevention strategy. I have now retired as a psychiatrist but continue with my registration. I am an Integrative Clinical Psychotherapist with special interest in treating patients with psychotherapy for PTSD, CPTSD (complex PTSD) and anxiety disorders, depression and Personality Disorders. I have a special interest in Integrative Clinical work and this work is in Integrating the techniques or lines of therapy.

I abide by the principles of purpose orientation and alignment-based approach to increase the effectiveness towards cohesion, which will be long lasting. This can be achieved by methodical and systematic processing.

I have over 40 years of experience working as a doctor of medicine. I am highly experienced having completed 36 years in psychiatry and thoracic medicine for 8 years.

Other areas of experience include industrial medicine, surgery, family practice and pathology.

I Assisted in a number of research clinical trials into Dementia and Depression, and was a Co-investigator in efficacy and toxicity study of a selective 5HT re uptake inhibitor antidepressant.

I Assisted in non-commercial clinical trials into tuberculosis in India. In India I was a Tutor in Pathology teaching Pathology to third year medical students; giving lectures in tuberculosis for Registered Nurses.

When I moved to England, I gave lectures on various topics in Psychiatry for Social Workers, Nurses and Care Workers. By invitation from the Alzheimer's Disease Society and Carers' Support Group, I have given talks on Dementia to carers at Pinehill Day Centre at St Leonards on Sea, East Sussex. A number of lectures/presentations have been given for medical colleagues on psychiatry and psychotherapy topics.

I have been a Long-term locum Consultant Psychiatrist for 8 years at St Anne's Centre, Department of Mental Health for the Elderly, with special interest in psychotherapy and qualified in Cognitive Behaviour Therapy. I Trained the staff at St Anne's Centre in Cognitive Behaviour Therapy, conducted 6 months duration of Foundation Course for CBT once a week for a few years.

I have also Worked as an independent psychiatrist and psychotherapist and continued to perform duties (on-call) as an approved Section 12(2) Medical Practitioner under the Mental Health Act 1983 (as amended 2007) and fulfilling annual conditions to continue to hold the licence.

I am a Senior BABCP accredited clinical psychotherapist. I continue to be an independent and integrative Clinical CBT therapist.

As honorary Fellow of Royal Society of Public Health and psychotherapist I am interested and became ambitious to write easily understandable self-help books for mental well-being and relapse prevention..

I recently obtained a diploma in EMDR.

I completed a number of presentations including:

1. Introduction to CBT
2. Medical overview of dementia.
3. Choline esterase inhibitors.
4. A rapid and methodical interpretation of ECG (emphasis made on prolonged QT interval as adverse effect due to psychotropic medication).
5. Therapeutic relationship.

6. 'Preliminary communication'. An epoch making publication by Freud and Breuer 1893 and 1895 on psychical mechanisms of hysterical symptoms

7. CBT for marital discord.

8. Hepatitis 'C' virus infection and the role of psychiatrists in the integrative approach of treating patients.

9. Transference and Countertransference.

10. Understanding the origins and development of Borderline Processes.

11. Understanding motivational interviewing.

12. Anti NMDA (n-Methyl D-Aspartate) receptor encephalitis and the significance of diverse presentation of this disorder with psychiatric symptomatology.

13. Stress management.

14. Deliberate self-harm.

15. Internal working models in attachment.

16. Standardisation of Mental Health Act assessments and procedures.

This is an exhaustive list of my attributes and hopefully gives credence to my understanding of the field of psychiatry and psychotherapy in relation to my competency in writing this book on The Integrative Technique of Relaxation in Relaxation Therapy.

Dr C.B.Ramachander

Relaxation Definition:

Relaxation is a state of being calm and composed, easing up in general restoring to a state of equilibrium of mind a body.

Integration – leading to innovation

The integrations are used in strategies and in many other major forms of lines of therapies. In integrating the techniques or lines of therapy, the aim of the therapy should be purpose orientated, and alignment based to increase the effectiveness which will be long standing. This can be achieved by methodical approaches navigating towards cohesiveness.

Integrative Relaxation Technique

There are many relaxation therapies particular forms of techniques. Most of them are effective if they are properly programmed and practised. However, the effectiveness is naturally short lived in the sense of duration of the time it can last if applying the usual methods.

The Innovative Integration of SLOW DEEP BREATHING which stimulates the parasympathetic nervous system with suggestion techniques, the effect is navigated towards cohesiveness.

I have found this particular type of integration, fulfils this need.

If the integration is practiced on a regular basis, the achievement is successful.

The Autonomic Nervous System and Psychophysiology of SDB

The psychophysiology of SLOW DEEP BREATHING and the amazing power of enhancement of the effect by integrative methods of self-suggestion techniques, creates positive changes in the individual which enhances and sustains modification in personality as relaxing the person and lifestyle changes occur towards calmness.

This technique has been found to be effective in treating Anxiety Disorders, Anxiety Depression, and as an important concomitant treatment for PTSD.

Psychophysiology of SLOW DEEP BREATHING by diaphragmatic breathing the following changes take place.

The contraction of the diaphragm muscle.

Diaphragm is innervated by the phrenic nerve which is stimulated – The contraction of the diaphragm facilitates expansion of the chest and increases oxygenation.

This causes stimulation of the parasympathetic nerve of the autonomic nervous system which is responsible for relaxation.

The autonomic nervous system is divided into two parts, the sympathetic nervous system and parasympathetic nervous system, and they supply the same organs and structures. E.g cardiac muscle, most glands and all smooth muscles.

They have antagonistic actions to each other. The sympathetic causes stimulation of the structures supplied E.g. Heart muscle causes increased pulse rate whereas the parasympathetic stimulation slows it down. Sympathetic stimulation causes dilation of the pupils and parasympathetic causes constriction of the pupils. The process of functioning can be described as the water tap system in balancing.

The two systems constantly discharge to the structures they supply.

Sympathetic stimulation causes excitatory effect and parasympathetic causes relaxing effect.

Sympathetic Nervous System

In stress reactions and stressful situations, the sympathetic nervous system dominates (Physical and psychological) the body automatically reacts to preparing for fight or flight. This leads to muscles getting tensed. There is a requirement for increased oxygen, use of more energy leads to catabolism. Breathing becomes faster, heart rate increases, the arteries to the peripheral parts of the body constrict, shunting more blood to the muscles which are active leading to the skin becoming cold. The pupils dilate and skin sweating occurs.

Parasympathetic nervous system.

This system is also based on the neuron pathway consisting of preganglionic and postganglionic neurons. The parasympathetic nervous system is most active when during relaxed periods, the heart rate slows down peristalsis and digestive system functioning are active, the pupils constrict, respiratory rate reduced, pupils constrict, and the person feels relaxed which is an anabolic process.

Sympathetic activity is adrenergic and parasympathetic activity is cholinergic.

Hormonal effects of hormonal health thro' parasympathetic nervous system which leads to decreased cortisol levels improving the hormonal balance. Slow deep breathing also improves the circulation leading to transport of hormones throughout the body while stimulation of the Vagus nerve takes place supporting relaxation and well-being.

The oxygenation levels improve, expands lung capacity followed by improved gas exchange. It widens vasodilation improving the blood circulation and lowers the blood pressure.

It reduces the body's response to stress in emotional regulation.

Improved oxygenation leads to stronger immune system.

Cognitive benefits of the slow deep breathing in the relaxation technique resulting in stimulation of parasympathetic nervous system include:

1. Increased ability to focus

2. Decreased rumination of thoughts

3. Improved balanced arousal levels

4. More positive emotions

5. Decreased emotional reactivity

By synchronising the heart rate, the brain releases endorphins leading to calming effect and mood lifting.

Integrative Technique of Relaxation

The Process: Relax in 5 steps to feel good.

Before starting, sit in a comfortable chair and close your eyes and smile genuinely.

1. Deep Breathing

- Inhale

Take slow deep breath without straining say ca….lm in your mind.

- Hold
- Exhale

Slowly breathe out completely. Say "Re……. laxed" in your mind.

- Do it 5-8 times – 2 or 3 sets

Follow this with the next step.

2. Autogenic Muscular Relaxation

Self generated muscle relaxation of the whole body.

The mechanism of generating relaxation by thinking. Relax each part of your body muscles. Start from the feet muscles and go up.

'Muscles in my feet are relaxing this sensation of wonderful feeling is now going to my ankles- now the legs → knees → thighs, pelvic muscles →lower abdomen → upper abdomen → chest- front of my neck → chin-facial muscles → forehead → top of my head → sides of my head → back of my head → back of my neck → upper back → shoulders → mid back → lower back muscle'

All the muscles in my whole body are relaxed and I feel wonderful.

Stay relaxed in your muscles for few minutes

3. Relax Your Mind By Thinking Relaxed

- My mind is relaxed.
- Stay relaxed by thinking relaxed.
- Thoughts are very powerful!

4. Visualisation

- Reliving of a peaceful and relaxing scenic atmosphere that you have experienced.
- The reliving is not the same as imagining.
- You have to re-experience during the session in reality.

Stay visulaising for a while, while you are deeply relaxed.

5. Autosuggestion of Positive Self Statements

In your deeply relaxed state suggest to yourself in your mind positive self statements which will remain in your subconscious, ready to achieve and happen.

Positive Self Affirmations Statement

They should be affirmative.

The pain has vanished

I feel lifted in my mood

I am able to walk now

I can finish this project with ease

The 5 steps are systematically arranged and they are in sequential order. When you open your eyes slowly, you will 'feel good' and relaxed.

As per the feedback I have received from my clients, this technique is powerful and effective.

Please start doing the relaxation technique twice daily.

Practice and Practice

Conclusion

The symptoms of anxiety will vanish if it is practiced regularly. Your mood gets lifted, your concentration improves, you are bound to feel good. The lifestyle changes to positive mode.

Dr C.B.Ramachander